YOUR KNOWLEDGE HAS VALUE

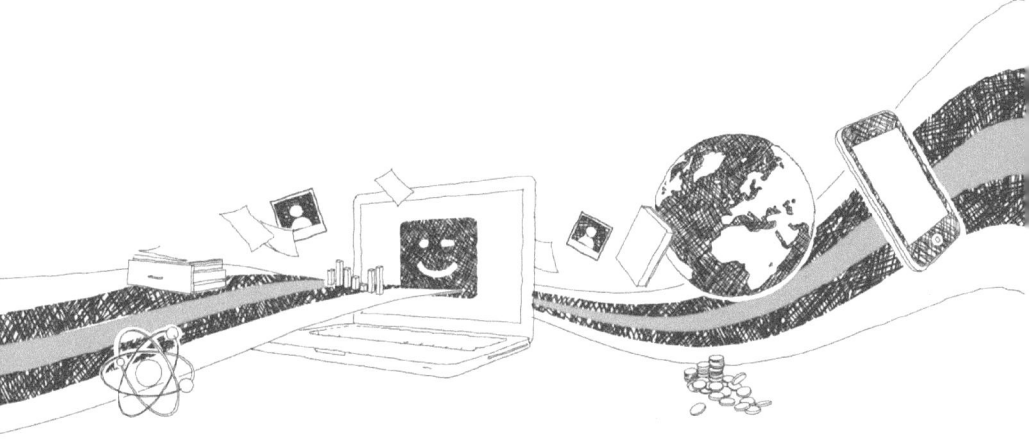

AF131213

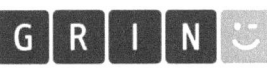

Bibliographic information published by the German National Library:

The German National Library lists this publication in the National Bibliography; detailed bibliographic data are available on the Internet at http://dnb.dnb.de .

Imprint:

Copyright © 2016 GRIN Verlag, Open Publishing GmbH
Print and binding: Books on Demand GmbH, Norderstedt Germany
ISBN: 9783668251717

This book at GRIN:

http://www.grin.com/en/e-book/321651/health-and-safety-in-the-construction-industry-the-effect-of-general-procurement

John Peter Cooney

Health and Safety in the Construction Industry. The effect of general Procurement and HSE Legislation on Construction Contractors and Employees

GRIN Publishing

GRIN - Your knowledge has value

Since its foundation in 1998, GRIN has specialized in publishing academic texts by students, college teachers and other academics as e-book and printed book. The website www.grin.com is an ideal platform for presenting term papers, final papers, scientific essays, dissertations and specialist books.

Visit us on the internet:

http://www.grin.com/

http://www.facebook.com/grincom

http://www.twitter.com/grin_com

HEALTH AND SAFETY IN THE CONSTRUCTION INDUSTRY: AN OVERVIEW OF THE EFFECT OF GENERAL PROCUREMENT AND HSE LEGISLATION ON CONSTRUCTION CONTACTORS AND EMPLOYEES

SUBMITTED: April 2016

John Peter Cooney, M.Phil Candidate,

School of the Built Environment, University of Salford;

SUMMARY: The management of health and safety is an issue that is relevant and crucial to all organisations across all industries, to include traditional industries, commercial, information technology (IT), the National Health Services (NHS), care homes, schools, higher educational institutions, travel and leisure, etc. Health and safety is specifically significant and crucial for the construction industry. In the United Kingdom, the construction industry is the largest of all industries. It accounts for about 8% of gross domestic product, employs about 10% of the national workforce and generates an annual turnover of up to £250 billion. The UK construction industry has a global reputation for the quality of its work and yet it remains one of the most dangerous industries in the nation .The research is based on a strategic approach to dealing with three major issues with regards to health and safety in the construction industry. First, the paper will identify and deal with the problem of how to improve organisational health and safety (OHS) through the monitoring of the process of procurement in construction projects. For instance, there is a strong belief in the construction industry that any organisational culture of any bidder chosen for a particular project will have an influence on the entire project. Hence, there is a need for the contractor to properly scrutinize bidders with regards to how they handle OHS and how this reflects on their organisational culture. In addition to the proper scrutiny of a client's OHS record, there is also an issue of financial and legal status of a client with regards to indemnity or any insurance considerations in the case of construction accidents. That is, can a client be held accountable for an accident? What type of accidents that will happen during work on the project that the client will be accountable for? Secondly, this paper will address the issue of cost-effectiveness in construction projects and how OHS is dealt with simultaneously. For instance, in the process of choosing a bidder, sometimes contractors may tend to ignore health and safety issues and decide to choose a client that will result in cost savings, or choosing the highest bidder irrespective of OHS concerns. Hence, there is a risk management concern to be dealt with in such cases. Third, the paper considers what type of strategic decisions and the responsibilities of both the contractor as well as the client in terms of dealing with OHS with regards to construction projects.

KEYWORDS: *NHS, OHS, construction, finance, health & safety, bidder, cost, risk, management, strategy.*

Table of Contents

1. INTRODUCTION

While the figures for the number of work related injuries in the construction industry have been steadily dropping since 2010/11, when 50 workers were fatally injured in 2014/15 where 35 workers died as a result of work related accidents (Health and Safety Executive, 2015), the economic costs still add up to about £500 million and 1.7 million working days lost due to work-related injuries and ill-health (Health and Safety Executive, 2015).

1.1 OVERVIEW

Health and safety is very important to all areas in the building/ construction industry. It has always been considered very important as it is considered to be a greatly exposed sector when it comes to occupational accidents. Indeed, improvements have been made in health and safety performance in some aspects of the construction industry, very little attention has been given to how the process of procurement impacts within the industry, with underlying themes of financial and legal liabilities and accountability for accidents. This has been seen in most countries – the reality is that the construction industry continually has injury and fatality statistics that make it one of the most dangerous industries in which to work predominantly, and how these statistics bear up within the organisational culture. Cutting corners, to deliver a project on time and to forego any relevant health and safety legislation, indeed to win a contract illegally, within the jurastiction, is becoming a concern. In view of this and as a result of the increasing number of accidents, the development and publication of standards and good engineering practices based on experience and codes started. In the UK for example, the required documentation is published in accessible outlets and forms such like official governmental publications, laws, directives and in standards, such as Health and Safety at Work Acts (HSWA, 1974). The principle aim of this paper is to give a general overview of the current state of health and safety in the construction industry, and to discuss the procurement, monitoring, cost effectiveness and strategy. It will explore methods used by stakeholders in the construction industry in terms of improving OHS, it will look into various aspects of these strategies, to include those to improve OHS through procurement, the economic priority of these strategies and the various responsibilities and duties of the stakeholders involved in the industry in terms of designing and implementing strategies that improve OHS

2. LITERATURE REVIEW - GENERAL DOCUMENTATION AND SOURCES FOR RESEARCH

Research into effectiveness of HSE programs and best practices are relatively plentiful. This paper will focus on reports,studies and other sources that examine the UK construction industry or are otherwise most relevant to conditions in the UK. The Health and Safety executive releases yearly statistics on construction work place injuries and their economic implications. Their yearly publications can be compared to understand the trends in workplace injury and illness numbers. The Statistics For Workplace Injuries in Construction reports also give figures for specific economic costs like healthcare losses and productivity losses due to injuries and illnesses.

2.1 STATISTICS FOR WORKPLACE INJURIES IN CONSTRUCTION WITHIN THE UK

A report published by HSE in 2014 revealed that about 69,000 cases are reported in the construction sector pertaining to work related illnesses in the UK. Of these around 64% relate to musculo-skeletal disorders. The report further highlighted the fact that around 3% of total workers in the sector sustain injuries such as slips, trips and fall, lifting and handling, falls from height, and being struck by object. These injuries have led to loss of 0.5 million working days for the companies in the country. The loss in working hours due to injuries in the sector is in addition to the loss of 1.2 million working days due to work related illnesses.

2.2 INDEPENDANT REPORT CRITICALLY EXAMINING CURRENT RULES AND SHORTCOMINGS OF THESE RULES (INCLUDES PROBLEMS WITH OVER-REGULATION)

An independent report published in 2011 examined shortcomings of the current health and safety rules and regulations. The report examined about 200 regulations and 53 approved codes of practices of HSE. It was found that the main problem is not with the rules and codes per se, but the way that they are implemented. There are inconsistencies in the way that regulators enforce health and safety rules. Moreover, the problem is also sometimes caused due to influence of the third parties that focus on unnecessary paperwork or go above the regulatory requirements when implementing workplace safety rules in the company. Lastly, there are some problems with some of the safety rules themselves in that they lack clarity, structure, and in some cases application.

2.3 HOW USING A COST BENEFIT ANALYSIS MODEL CAN HELP REDUCE WORKPLACE INJURIES

Another pertinent issue relating to workplace safety and health in the construction sector is that there has not been any significant focus on conducting cost benefit analysis (CBA) of activities to help prevent accidents at the workplace. A research study surveyed 79 contractors to find out their view on whether the benefits outweigh costs involved in accident prevention actions. It was found that the benefit to cost ration according to contractors as 3:1. Using a CBA analysis model can help influence the decision making process that relates to preventing accidents and injuries at the workplace.

2.4 SUGGESTIONS FOR SPECIFIC COST BENEFIT ANALYSIS MODELS TO ASSESS COSTS OF ACCIDENTS TO CONTRACTORS

The HSE had introduced an on line interactive tools in 2005 for the contractors to evaluate associated costs of accidents for the company. That said, the online tool did not offer sufficient details to properly gauge the true costs of accidents. Companies need to be provided with an effective CBA framework that helps them better manage health and safety issues. The framework should include such tools as net present value (NPV) and willingness to pay (WTP) that will better help decision makers in assessing outcome of different strategies, and thereby make decisions in a structured manner.

2.5 REPORT CONCERNING BEST PARACTICES IN PROCUREMENT TO DECREASE ACCIDENTS

Institute of Civil Engineers (ICE) had published a report in which they highlighted best practices to prevent workplace accidents. The report stated that workplaces accidents and injuries can be prevented by focusing on health and safety during procurement of construction related services and works. Companies need to ensure that the contract terms on which services are procured comply with work and safety legislations. Subcontractors must be chosen based on the criteria of adhering to health and safety regulations, and not on the basis of price alone.

2.6 STUDIES ON OHS ISSUES IN WORKPLACE AND CREATING INTERVENTION STRATAGIES.

In 2007, HSE had analyzed health and safety issues relating to procurements in the construction sector. The report surveyed public sector clients and private sector suppliers. It was found that only some of the public sector clients performed well when it came to meeting health and safety obligation. There is a lot that needs to be done to embed safety and health responsibilities with the procurements process.

HSE conducted similar survey two years later in 2009 and found that respondents feel little progress has been made during the intervening period in this regard. Most of the respondents stated that there needs to be significant improvement on how the public sector clients fulfil their responsibilities related to health and safety during the procurement process.

2.7 STUDY ON HOW WORKERS ARE AFFECTED BY HSE REGULATIONS

A number of factors have been identified by research scholars that influence attitudes regarding safety at the construction sites. Langford, Rowlinson, and Sawacha studied attitudes using a research model that linked safety management implementation strategies, attitudes of workers about safety, and behavioural factors displayed by the workers at site. The study was able to identify 56 variables that directly influences attitude of the workers towards safety. Of these five factors were found to have a major influence on safety attitudes that include industry norms and culture, organizing for safety supervision and equipment management, management behaviour, and risk taking attitude of the workers.

2.8 DISCUSSION ON CONTRACTOR SELECTION METHODS

Contractors should be selected carefully by using effective selecting modelling methods. These include Multi-attribute analysis, Bespoke approaches, Cluster analysis, and Multivariate discriminant analysis, Multi-attribute utility theory. Multiple regression, and Fuzzy set theory.

2.9 LEXIS NEXIS RESOURCES ON LEGAL IMPLICATIONS OF WORKPLACE INJURIES

There are legal implications for the companies of workplace related injuries. UK laws states that a claimant can sue the company in court and receive compensation if it is proved that (1) the company had a duty of care, (2) there was some business relationship with the party, (3) the injury incurred by the claimant was foreseeable, and (4) it is just, fair, and reasonable to impose the duty of care.

2.10 MIT MODEL FOR STRATEGIC DECISIONS FOR STAKEHOLDERS AND CONTRACTORS

The legal complications and other costs attached with workplace injury necessitates the need for implementing tool to assess and lessen the risk of injury at the workplace. One such tool that has been suggested by scholars that can help companies to integrate OHS risk management in the process is ToolSHed that has been currently being tested in the Australian construction industry. It is an innovative decision support and information management tool that relies on a web-based architecture to offer support through knowledge acquisition and work process modelling.

2.11 HSE IMPLICATIONS IN THE DESIGN STAGE

A number of studies looked at the implications of health and safety during the design stage. It has been found that decisions that are made upstream from the construction site greatly influence worker safety. A definite link has been found between design for construction safety and fatalities at the site. In fact, a study had found around 224 fatalities that were somehow related to inefficient workplace safety design.

This shows important role of designers in ensuring safety at the construction site. A study has found that designers play an important role especially during the initial stage of the projects. The importance of construction contractors increases during the middle and final leg of the project. This is contrary to the common view that construction contractors are solely responsible for safety at the workplace. In the US, for instance, only one third of design firms stated that they made design decisions based on safety conditions at the workplace.

2.12 DECISIONS FOR STAKEHOLDERS

Construction companies are recommended to select contractors based on multi attribute analysis technique and prequalification criteria using weightings to mirror the importance of the respective criteria. The goal according to some scholars should be to select the most suitable contractor that is able to deliver the project while ensuring the best value for money. Note that the selection should be based on the best value for money and not price. This is possible by implementing fuzzy decision model that takes into account multiple criteria for selection of construction clients, relationship among decision criteria, and preferences of construction clients relating to criteria for selecting the contractor.

3. MONITORING OF PROCUREMENT

Unlike many other industries that are involved in mass production, the construction industry tends to focus on one-prototype projects (Sabol, 2007). However, according to Lenzen and Lundie (2012) there are certain comparisons to be made between construction and mass products: cases where a prototype from construction emerges as a model, and this model in turn is then replicated. Also, unlike the case of mass production, in construction the client is normally the one that takes the initiative in having the constructions designed and build (More and Joshi, 2014). In such as a case, the client pays for the construction and remains the actor (More and Joshi, 2014). The client is the one that places the order for the construction - hence he may sell or even let the construction for a later period (More and Joshi, 2014). And in all construction projects, there are different types of clients: those involved in one-off requirements

(Takim, 2008), organisations involved in a regular process of development, as well those with huge development programmes that tend to employ technically skilled staff (International Labour Organisation, 2001). So, as the clients take the initiative in placing an order for a construction project, the contractors and other industry consultants on the other hand work on the continuous process of developing markets for their products and services (Rundquist *et al.*, 2013). This comes with the development of certain private to public partnership models that involve a process of pre-financing the initial costs of construction to the client. Contractors and consultants are also often involved in trying to convince potential clients through the provision of feasibility studies for upcoming projects as well free costs (Vadnjal, 2011; Stroe, 2013).Some studies have tried to identify a procurement path,for example, (Smith e*t al.*, 2004; Babatunde, Opawole and Ujaddughe, 2010). Such a path involves the client trying to engage the private sector for various construction activities, such as conducting feasibility studies, design, building, operation, and maintenance (Smith *et al.*, 2004). The client therefore has the onus of defining a procurement path. Hence according to Miller et al. (2009) depending on the in-house capabilities, knowledge and understanding of the construction process itself, as well as the client's demands, the client must define a procurement path. However, Janak (2010) states that the most common form of procurement for all construction contracts is general contracting. In this regard, the client engages a team of designers; such a team designs the product to be built; and then the design team, on behalf of the client, engages the services of the contractor who only has a relationship with the design team. However, Hagstedt and Thideman (2013) in their Master's thesis, they state that such a model is only useful in the case of simple and straightforward construction projects. Nowadays, many construction projects require multidisciplinary skills during the design phase. The design team often needs the support of specialists. Hence, the design team may have to procure the services of specialists such as subcontractors and advisors. This kind of model is one recommended by O'Brien, Soibelman and Elvin (2003). However, according to Sacks et al. (2015) the problem with such a model is that the design team will have to coordinate the inputs of the various advisors to the construction project. Therefore, as Sacks et al. (2015) state a lack of coordination will often lead to a mismatching of design inputs and that of construction inputs. Most often the contractor has a responsibility of filling in or adjusting the design that was provided by the design team. In addition to this, according to Sacks et al. (2015) the contractor will also have to plan delivery of inputs. The procurement time of some specialist equipment may normally take a long time - such as the entire construction process. Hence there is a need to procure the services of subcontractors well ahead of the commencement of the project (Clegg, Kornberger and Pitsis, 2011).

3.1. Strategy

A "strategic" point of view of an inventory network idea was developed in the 1980s which in this way advanced into strategic procurement (Porter, 1985; Christopher,1992; Lamming, 1992; Lamming and Cox, 1995; Ross, 1998). Regularly this included situating such a method intensely in the commercial area by creating proper sourcing and administration methodologies for suppliers. Porter (1985) built up the idea of a "value chain" as an apparatus to enhance aggressive advantage in an industry.In addition, the idea of key acquirement organization, which is the progression of an outside sourcing and supply method planned to keep up a reasonable position for that organisation, in regards to procurement Lamming (1995), identified the significance of supplier advancement through united business associates and vital strategic community oriented organizations to empower an enhanced production within the company to occur. He termed this lean supply. Lamming likewise suggested that fulfilling a lean method technique is a matter in perspective of the method for competition in business areas, in light of the way that the suppliers are incorporated in the meantime in a couple of other distinctive chains Strategic procurement is much more extensive than the lean development. It is an idea relevant to architectural, engineering and construction disciplines. An important part of strategic procurement can be seen with the co-operation of multiple companies, and as such has developed since the 1980's as such collaborations have indeed developed in one business after another (Gomes-Casseres, 1996).

Ross (1998), recognized and suggests two levels in conceptualizing production network administration, to be specific the strategic and tactical, his examination focused on the rising vital abilities of the production network administration idea. He states that, quote - "Procurement management is a continuously evolving management philosophy that seeks to unify the collective productive competencies and resources of the business functions found both within the enterprise and outside in the allied business partners located along intersecting supply channels into a highly competitive, customer-enriching supply system focused on developing innovative solutions and synchronizing the of marketplace products,services and information to create unique, individualized sources of customer value". However, procurement issues, within the AEC area, does lead and can produce traits for the unscrupulous, to obtain an advantage over other rival companies in the need to seek contracts.

4. VETTING BIDDERS FOR CONTRACTS

Under the current Health and Safety laws in the UK, both the client and the contractor have responsibilities to reduce the risk of work-related injuries and illness. Clients need to develop and deliver a clear policy in regards to the HS standards they expect from contractors. This policy needs to be well publicised so that agents on the client side like procuring officers and contractor side like the tendering officers understand the priorities of the client (Wells and Hawkins, 2013). The clients should also have realistic expectations in terms of health and safety and this can be achieved with a survey of the market and making sure that the criteria they are setting can be met by the available market. This analysis of the market should include the OHS regulatory framework already set in the market and a study of the common OHS strategies used by contractors in the market.

In the past few years, there has been an increase in the risk models that contractors can use during the bidding process to allocate risk contingencies. Some of the risk models that have been introduced for assessing risks include influence diagramming based technique (Al-Bahar and Crandall, 1990), fuzzy set model (Tah et al., 1993; Paek et al., 1993; and Zeng et al., 2007), and logic based ANN model (Liu and Lang, 2005). However, most of the recent research studies have shed light to the fact that the risk assessment tools are not commonly used by the contractors. Only seven contractors in UK were found by Tah et al. (1994) to have used risk assessment tools to assess the risks during the bidding process. Moreover, Akintoye and MacLeod (1997) and Norman, 1993; etc.). Capital market and portfolio theories state that there are two types of risks present in the market (Fisher and Jordan, 1996). The first is the systematic risk that is outside the control of the organizations such as interest rate and market risk, purchasing power risk, and natural calamities. The second type of risk is the unsystematic risk that is inherent to organization and can be controlled. It includes financial and business risk. Both these risks are also relevant to the construction sector according to Dorfam (2002) and Tah et al. (1993).Fisher and Jordan (1996) state that one way of estimating the price that meets the profit target is through quantifying the risk and setting a required rate of return. The rate of return takes into account a risk free rate and also compensation of the individual risk factors. Connoly (2006) said that the risk element contains costs that in some cases can be catastrophic. But estimating the price risk is not that easy as has been revealed in a survey of 400 top contractors in the US (Mochtar and Arditi, 2001).

Mulholland and Christian (1999) conducted a conceptual study in which an analytical approach was taken to assess the risk in the construction projects. It was found that projects that are undertaken in dynamic and multifaceted environment results in high risks and uncertainty that is compounded by the time constraints. Flanagan and Norman (1993) say that every construction project has some unique features and risks. On the other hand, Wright and Ayton (1994) are of the view that risks are not unique in the sector. Hughes and Hillebrand (1985), state that there are a number of factors that makes the construction industry unique. They are of the view that the there are a number of factors that are contractual, economic, environment, and political in nature all affect how construction work is awarded, reported, and described. Some of the factors outlined by the authors that affect construction sector include competitive tendering, production, preliminary expenses, low fixed capital requirements, tendency to operate with low working capital, delays to cash inflow, government interventions, seasonal fluctuations and effects, and uncertain weather conditions, unpredictable ground conditions, and no long term guarantees or performance liability.

5. STRATEGIC DECISIONS IN CONSTRUCTION PROJECTS

It is important to consider health and safety issues through the entirety of a project, from planning and design to construction and evaluation. This will not only reduce costs but improve productivity through better predictive capabilities and management of operational and production costs. Proper integration of Health and Safety strategies into the processes will also allow for innovations in the design and construction processes of the project (WorkSafe Victoria, 2010).Contractors undertake the construction project using a team comprising of different department. Most of the contributors make decisions that affect health and safety at the worksite. In some cases, the project team consists of external members such as advocacy groups or regulatory agencies. It is important that the construction company identify health and safety issues relates to the sector during the decision making process. A construction company should understand interests of all the stakeholders and establish proper processes while complying with the highest quality health and safety standards that are specific to the sector. The company should make sure that decisions made in response to interests of the stakeholders are consistent with the OHS standards.

The supply chain in the construction industry is fragmented with very little communication taking place between the individuals that initiate, manufacture, design, utilize, and/or maintain the facilities. Lack of communication between different team members can prevent establishment of shared goals and objectives that will negatively affect health and safety at the organization level. Poor communication and the formal distance between the construction and the design department is especially identified as a major barrier to implementation of effective

11

health and safety procedures within the organization. It has also been linked with higher incidence of fatalities at the construction worksite. As compared to other department, constructors have a deep understanding of the processes mainly due to specialized knowledge, training and expertise of the individuals. Moreover, they are directly responsible for the project outcomes. As a result, they usually have a greater interest and motivation in ensuring the work is performed safely with minimum safety and health risk for the workers. They can provide advice to the decision makers about OHS before the start of the construction process. When they fed knowledge about the construction process 'upstream' at the initial phase of the construction project, it will result in better decision making with greater chances of health and safety risks being reduced eliminated completely at the source

6. FINANCIAL AND LEGAL IMPLICATIONS WITH CONSTRUCTION ACCIDENTS

There are several pieces of legislation relevant to workplace injuries and accidents in the UK. The first concerns reporting and is called the Reporting of Injuries, Diseases and Dangerous Occurences Regulation (RIDDOR) and was enacted in 2013. The regulations state that employers and people in control of the workplace are responsible to report the included accidents, diseases and any dangerous occurrences. In the UK, the Health and Safety Executive monitors and enforces health and safety laws and regulations. There are several pieces of legislation relevant to workplace injuries and accidents in the UK. The first concerns reporting and is called the Reporting of Injuries, Diseases and Dangerous Occurences Regulation (RIDDOR) and was enacted in 2013. The regulations state that employers and people in control of the workplace are responsible to report the included accidents, diseases and any dangerous occurrences. In the UK, the Health and Safety Executive monitors and enforces health and safety laws and regulations. The construction sector plays a major role in the economic development of almost every country in the world. That being said, the work involved in construction is regarded as the most hazardous as compared to other industrial activities. Injuries incurred while performing construction work is about 50% higher as compared to all other work (Schneider, 2001). The risk of musculo-skeletal injury is especially higher among construction workers. Accidents and mishaps at the construction sites results in injury and/or death of many worker every years. That is why it is of fundamental importance for the construction company to assess the risk at the work site, and take effective measures to minimize the risk. Through continuous monitoring and surveillance, the work related injury risk can be minimized (Odetoyinbo, 1986). According to Lucy et al (1999), work related accidents are unexpected and unplanned occurrences that results in loss of productivity due to disturbance in the planned work sequence, injury, and damage to the plant and equipment that interrupts normal flow of production. O.S.H.A (2005) reports that about 60,000 deaths occur every year around the world due to mishaps at the construction sites, and the rate of fatalities in the sector is much higher as compared to others. A study conducted by Jaselskis and Suazo (1994) showed that most of these accidents occur due lack of commitment to workplace safety.

7. COST EFFECTIVENESS

Compromising on health and safety for short term cost benefits when designing HS strategies is not always beneficial. Any cost-benefit analysis done on the project should take into account the risk of injuries and illnesses and their expected costs when adjusted for risk. Most models predict that making decisions after factoring in possible costs from injuries and illnesses will show that greater priority on health and safety results in cost savings. Industrial and academic model creation tools like including multi-variate analysis, fuzzy set theory and multiple regressions can all be used to create an optimal model that takes into account HS considerations. According to Baccarini (1999) the success of a project is synonym to effectiveness. In other words the degree of achievement of project goals determines its effectiveness. Project team is formed to achieve and accomplish goals and the success of the project is determine how well those goals have been achieved. The top project priorities include completing the project on time, within the budget, and meeting technical specifications and mission. This corroborates with findings of De wit (1988) who found that that success of the project depends on the achievement of project objectives relating to quality, cost, time, and mission. According to a number of researchers the success factor in the construction industry relates to *effectiveness* and *efficiency* measures (Atkinson, 1999; Belout, 1998; Crawford and Bryce, 2003; De Wit, 1988; Brudney and England, 1982; Pinto and Slevin, 1988:1989; and Smith, 1998).

The term efficiency refers to maximum output obtained by utilizing a given level of resources, while effectiveness refers to achievement of objects and goals relating to the project. Pinto and Slevin (1988:1989) say that both the *effectiveness* and *efficiency* measures determine success of the project. Efficiency measures relate to internal organizational structures and strong management such as adherence to budget and schedules, basic expectation regarding performance, etc. It can also be said that efficiency of a project relates to user satisfaction, meeting project goals and objectives. All the factors jointly play an important part in success of the project. A project that is completed within the budget, delivered on time, but does not conforms to user's requirement will not be confirmed a success. Project efficiency can only be achieved when the a standard methodology and system are out in place by the company management (George, 1968). This aligns with the findings of Nyhan and Martin (1999) and Smith (1998) who says that the efficiency of the project relates to effective utilization of human resource and equipment, while effectiveness relates to outcome of the project. Maloney (1990) suggest that the efficiency of projects in the construction sector depends on the effective utilization of resources. This may be represented by the ratio of resources required divided by the resources consumed. Effectiveness of the project, on the other hand, depends on the achievement of organization's objectives. Cameron and Whetton (1993) contributed to the knowledge of product effectiveness and efficiency by demonstrating that a system is effective only when the objectives of the project are achieved. Since most of the construction projects focus on client's needs, an effective project is one that effectively meets the needs of the client. Crawford and Bryce (2003) state that the success of the project is determined by evaluating effectiveness and efficacy of the project. Project efficiency or 'doing the things right' relates to process and cost efficiency. In other words, it refers to efficient conversion of inputs to the output while remaining within the schedule and budget. Efficiency also relate to evaluating project success based on the effectiveness and efficient utilization of financial, human, and natural resources. Effectiveness on the other hand refers to 'doing the right thing' is related with development of appropriateness and worthiness of the chosen project goal. A project may be executed efficiently or implemented ahead of cost and time schedules , but if the goals are not set right or that does not address the core vulnerabilities of the project it will not be considered a success. For this reason it is important to conduct a strong initial development problem analysis to ensure that the project goal address all the factors that will have a great bearing on the success of the project.

Atkinson (1999) suggests that measuring efficiency requires assessing project success based on project management process criteria. On the other hand, effectiveness means assessing the results or outcome of the system in terms of organizational benefits and achieving project goals. In lighting of the above discussion, it could be concluded that the success of the project depends on both the efficiency (project output) and effectiveness (project outcomes) that covers a wide area (Abdel-Razek, 1997; Atkinson, 1999; Cameron and Whetten 1993; Maloney, 1990; Mbugua, 2000; Nyhan and Martin 1999; Pinto and Slevin 1988:89; and Smith 1998). In view of this, the paper discusses and documents the analysis of factors that relate to effectiveness of a project in the construction sector in the eyes of four project stakeholders namely private clients, contractors, Government, and consultants.In the first stage of the study, we examined mean values of the responses and ranked them on the basis of importance. Afterwards a detailed comparison of ranking order was made between the different groups. The second stage of the study consisted of testing the hypothesis by using non parametric testing method known as Kruskal-Wallis One-Way ANOVA (Analysis of Variance) test for an independent sample. The purpose of the study was to analyze difference in the individuals' opinions relating to the individual factors among the four groups at a significance level of 5%. The mean ranking technique showed that all the variables were significant. However, this result is meaningless and superfluous. Therefore, we conducted factor analysis technique using principal component analysis (PCA) to test the effectiveness of the variables and identify main factors so as to gain deeper understanding of the factor group that underpin success of the project.

8. CONCLUSION

The overall findings from the paper conclude and highlight statistics to accidents and ill-health within the construction industry, and gives account of several parameters to enable and deduce practices regarding the monitoring of procurement, vetting bidders for contracts, strategic decisions, financial and legal implications with construction accidents and cost effectiveness. Initially, the literature reveals several factors of sources from other areas of commerce, indeed educational institutions such as MIT, who justify a software model that can offer support through knowledge acquisition and work process modelling. Construction companies have used this software for building development in a time coninuum, known as BIM, (Building Information Modelling), the knowledge acquisition element could prove useful in such a model.

The literature review depicts and highlights areas of importance to the effect of OHS. It suggests the importance of the correct implementation of rules and regulations and indicates drawbacks such as excessive paperwork, hence raising costs. It found also that organisations and companies in the public sector performed averagely when applying health & safety legislation, and also to suggest that a relatively few on-site employees knew about management implementation strategies.

It was found through the research that unlike many other industries that are involved, for example mass production, a company tends to focus on one particular product or project. This was confirmed to enable easier procurement methods, to then be replicated. Numerous methods can be attributed to good monitoring, as discussed – feasibility studies, developing markets particular to the product or build and the development of "in-house" techniques or methodologies for monitoring buyers. The introduction of strategy is discussed, thus bringing forward the idea of a "supply-chain" idealism, to give an aggressive advantage in the industry hence to evolve a clearer management philosophy and to create unique, individualised sources of customer value.

Risk models for vetting bidders for contracts have indeed increased over time, using specific set modelling such as diagramming techniques, fuzzy set modelling and logic based ANN models. The research suggests that contractors tend not to use such models, which further highlights that the award of a contract from the vetting process stems from contractural, economic, environmental and political – all have an effect. Other factors discussed to conclude no long term guarantees of performance or liability.

The attitude of health & safety to planning and design is also considered, highlighting and giving reason to improve costs through better predictions and management of operational and production costs. The research also deduces that very little communication takes place in the supply chain, hence the need for proper strategic decisions being able to be made and justified, within a health & safety overview in the organisation.

Financial and legal implication are seen also to be of a concern, and highlighted with the use of government publications, documentation and other sources. This being said, the construction industry does observe and recognises all such legislation, however much more has to be done. Cutting costs can also have a considerable effect on health & safety strategies, research suggests that a company showing greater respect for the legislation results in cost – saving. Its effectiveness is seen as the product of good management, the observation of good budget controls and a basic expectation of a good performance..

Cost effeciency would require a building or project success based on the project management system. It can be seen from this paper that many entities and parameters affect the general procurement and HSE legislation on construction contractors and employees, however further research would prove beneficial for the advancement and overview of contractor selection methods, strategy, monitoring of procurement, vetting bidders,financial implication and cost effectiveness, for subsequent development and understanding of points in the abstract.

9. REFERENCES

Abdel-Razek, R.H. (1997). How Construction Managers would like their Performance to be evaluated. *Journal of Construction Engineering and Management*, ASCE, **123**(3), pp.208-13

Akintoye, A. S. and MacLeod, J. M. (1997) Risk analysis and management in construction, *International Journal of Project Management*, 15(1), 31-38.

Al-Bahar, J. F. and Crandall, K. C. (1990) Systematic risk management approach for construction projects, *Journal of Construction Engineering and Management, ASCE.*

Atkinson, R. (1999). Project management: cost, time and quality, two best guesses and a phenomenon, its time to accept other success criteria. *International Journal of Project Management*, 17(6), pp. 337-342

Belout, A. (1998). Effects of human resource management on project effectiveness and success: towards a new conceptual framework. International Journal of Project Management, 16 (1), pp. 21-26

Brudney, J.L. and England, R.E. (1982). Urban policy making and subjective service evaluations: Are they compatible. *Public Administrative Review*, 42 (2), pp. 127-135.

Cameron, K.S., and Whetten, D.A. (1983). *Organisational Effectiveness: A Comparison of Multiple Models.* New York: Academic Press

Christopher, M. (1992) *Logistics and Supply Chain Management Strategies for Reducing Costs and Improving Services*,Pitman, London.

Connolly, J. P. (2006) Discussion of modeling a contractor"s markup estimation, *Journal of Construction Engineering and Management*, **132**(6), 657-658

Crawford, P. and Bryce, P. (2003). Project Monitoring and evaluation: a method for enhancing the efficiency and effectiveness of aid project implementation. *International Journal of Project Management*, pp. 363-373

De Wit, A. (1988). Measurement of project success. *Project management*, 6(3), pp. 164-170

Fischer, D. and Jordan, R. (1996) *Security analysis and portfolio management,* London: Prentice-Hall.

George, C.S. (1968). The History of Management Thought. Englewood Cliffs, N.J.*: Prentice-hall, Inc.*

Gomes-Casseres, B. (1997) *The Alliance Revolution: The New Shape of Business Rivalry*, Harvard University Press, Cambridge, MA

Hughes, W.P. (1998) Financial protection in the UK building industry: bonds, retentions and guarantees, London: Spon.

Hughes, W. P. and Hillebrandt, P.M. (2003) Construction industry: historical overview and technological change, In: Mokyr, Joel (ed.-in. chief) *The Oxford Encyclopaedia of Economic History*, Oxford: Oxford University Press, 2003, 1, 504-512.

Jaselskis E.J and Suazo, G.A.R (1994) a survey of construction site safety in Honduras. *Construction Management and economics* 12, 245-255.

Lamming, R. (1992) Supplier strategies in the automotive components industry: development towards lean production. Ph.D. thesis, University of Sussex.

Lamming, R. (1993) *Beyond Partnership: Strategies for Innovation and Lean Supply*, Prentice Hall, Englewood Cliffs, NJ.

Lamming, R. and Cox, A. (1995) *Strategic Procurement Management in the 1990s: Concepts and Cases*, Earlsgate Press, London.

Liu, A.M.M. and Leung, M. (2002). Developing a soft value management model. *International Journal of Project Management*, 20 (5), pp. 341-349

Lucy J.S, Ian J, Ian V. (1999). Increasing construction productivity through total loss control; *journal of R.I.C.S research foundation* COBRA, pg 266-276.

Mochtar, K. and Arditi, D. (2001) Pricing strategy in the US Construction industry, *Construction Management and Economics* 19, 405–415.

Nyhan, R.C., and Martin, L.L. (1999). Comparative performance measurement. *Public Productivity & Management Review*, 22(3), pp.348-64

O'Brien, B. (1995). Construction supply—chains: case study, integrated cost and performance analysis. In IGLC Annual Conference, Albuquerque, NM, available at http://cic. vtt.. /lean/conferences.htm

O'Brien, B. (1998) Capacity costing approaches for construction supply-chain management. Ph.D. thesis, Stanford University.

Odetoyinbo O.A (1986). The relevance of hazard assessment and control to practioneer accident. *Thesis On building construction site* pg 56, 61, 114.

Paek, J.H., Lee, Y.W. and Ock, J.H. (1993) Pricing construction risk: fuzzy set application, *Journal of Construction Engineering and Management ASCE*, **109**(4), 743-56.

Porter, M. (1985) *Competitive Advantage, Creating and Sustaining Superior Perfomance*, The Free Press, New York.

Pinto, J.K. and Slevin, D.P. (1994). The Project Implementation Profile: An International Perspective. In Cleland D.I

Smith, M. (1998). Measuring organisational effectiveness. *Management Accounting*, 76 (9), pp. 34-36.

YOUR KNOWLEDGE HAS VALUE

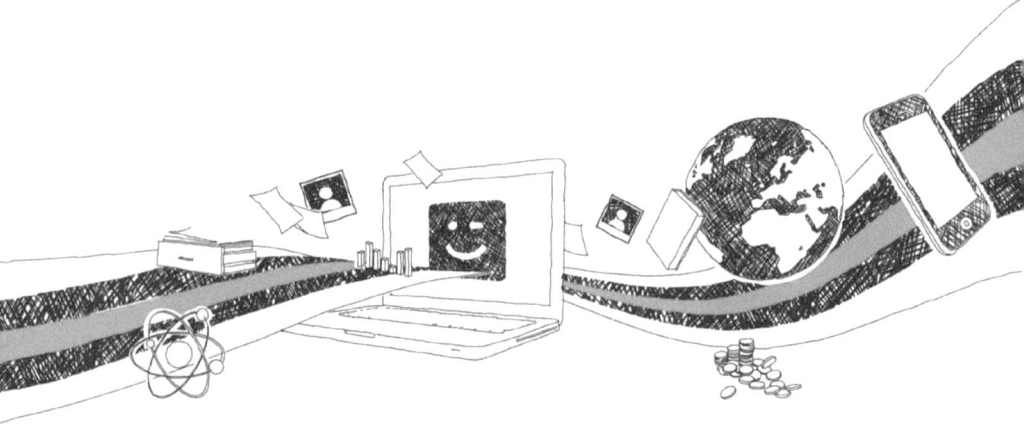

- We will publish your bachelor's and master's thesis, essays and papers

- Your own eBook and book - sold worldwide in all relevant shops

- Earn money with each sale

Upload your text at www.GRIN.com and publish for free

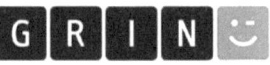